Understanding Chronic Lymphocytic Leukaemia

BACUP 3 Bath Place, Rivington Street, London, EC2A 3JR

BACUP was founded by Dr Vicky Clement-Jones, following her own experiences with ovarian cancer, and offers information, advice and emotional support to cancer patients and their families.

We produce publications on the main types of cancer, treatments, and ways of living with cancer. We also produce a newspaper, *BACUP News*, three times a year.

Our success depends on feedback from users of the service. We thank everyone, particularly patients and their families, whose advice has made this booklet possible.

Administration 071 696 9003

Cancer Information Service 071 613 2121

Freeline (outside London) 0800 181199

Counselling Service 071 696 9000 (London based)

British Association of Cancer United Patients and their families and friends. A company limited by guarantee. Registered in England and Wales company number 2803321. Charity registration number 1019719. Registered office as above.

Medical consultant: Maurice Slevin, MD, FRCP

Editor: Annie Jackson

Illustrations by Andrew Macdonald

Cover design by Malcolm Harvey Young

First published 1989, revised edition 1994

©BACUP 1989, 1993

Typeset and printed in Great Britain by Lithoflow Ltd., London

ISBN 1-870403-50-9

Contents

Introduction

This information booklet has been written to help you understand more about chronic lymphocytic leukaemia. We hope it answers some of the questions you may have about its diagnosis and treatment.

We can't advise you about the best treatment for yourself because this information can only come from your own doctor, who will be familiar with your full medical history.

At the end of this booklet you will find a list of other BACUP publications, some useful addresses and recommended books. If, after reading this booklet, you think it has helped you, do pass it on to any of your family and friends who might find it interesting. They too may want to be informed so they can help you cope with any problems you may have.

Blood cells

Leukaemia is a general term for cancer of the white blood cells. Blood is made in the bone marrow and contains:

red blood cells which contain haemoglobin to carry oxygen around the body

white blood cells which fight infections

platelets which help to prevent and stop bleeding.

There are two main types of white cell, neutrophils and lymphocytes, which work together to fight infection in the body. These cells circulate around the body in the blood; lymphocytes are also found in the lymph glands and in lymphatic channels, which are somewhat like veins, but instead of carrying blood, carry a clear fluid, lymph, from the tissues to the lymph glands.

The lymphatic system is part of the body's natural defences against infection. There are lymph glands in the neck, under the armpits, in each groin, and in the chest and abdomen. The tonsils, liver and the spleen (which breaks down old blood cells) also contain lymphatic tissue.

What is chronic lymphocytic leukaemia (CLL)?

Chronic lymphocytic leukaemia is a cancer of the lymphocytes. Production of white cells normally takes place in an orderly and controlled manner, but in leukaemia, the process gets out of control; the cells multiply too quickly producing too many white blood cells. Over a period of time the bone marrow progressively becomes replaced by 'bad cells' at the expense of the normal white cells, red cells and platelets. The disease usually progresses very slowly, hence the term 'chronic'.

Chronic lymphocytic leukaemia mainly affects older people and is rare in people under the age of 40.

There are three other main types of leukaemia: chronic myeloid leukaemia, acute lymphoblastic leukaemia and acute myeloblastic leukaemia. BACUP has separate booklets about these types.

What causes chronic lymphocytic leukaemia?

Although the cause of chronic lymphocytic leukaemia is unknown, research is going on all the time into possible causes of the disease.

Chronic lymphocytic leukaemia, like other cancers, is not infectious and cannot be passed on to other people.

What are the symptoms of chronic lymphocytic leukaemia?

Because the disease progresses slowly, it is difficult to detect in its early stages. Quite often, a person will have no symptoms and the disease may be discovered only when a blood test is taken for a different reason.

Some people go to see their doctor because they feel unusually tired or look pale due to a lack of red blood cells (anaemia).

Some people get frequent infections which may take a long time to get better. This is because of a shortage of neutrophils which are the cells that normally kill bacteria. Occasionally people may have problems with bleeding and bruising due to lack of platelets.

In addition to any of these symptoms the abnormal lymphocytes may collect in the lymph glands and cause painless swellings or the spleen may become enlarged and cause a tender lump in the upper half of the abdomen.

Sweating or fever at night can also sometimes occur. Some people lose weight.

If you do have any of the above symptoms, you must have them checked by your doctor, but remember, they are common to many illnesses other than chronic lymphocytic leukaemia. Most people with these symptoms do not have leukaemia.

How does the doctor make the diagnosis?

Your family doctor (General Practitioner) will examine you and do a blood test. Depending on the result, he or she will then refer you to a hospital for specialist advice and treatment.

The doctor at the hospital will take your full medical history, do a physical examination and further blood tests.

If these show leukaemia cells to be present, the hospital doctor will want to do a bone marrow test to be sure of the diagnosis and to plan the best treatment for you.

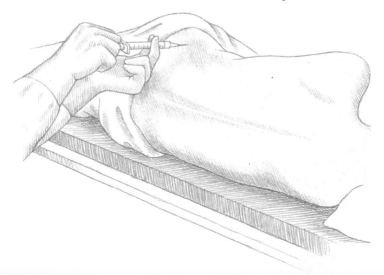

Bone marrow test

A small sample of bone marrow is taken from the hip bone (pelvis) or the breast bone (sternum), and looked at under the microscope to see if it contains any abnormal white blood cells. The doctor will be able to tell which type of leukaemia it is by identifying the type of abnormal white cell.

The bone marrow test is done under a local anaesthetic; you will be given a small injection to numb the area and a needle is passed gently through the skin into the bone. A tiny sample of the marrow is then drawn into a syringe.

The whole procedure takes about 15 minutes. You may experience some discomfort for a second or two as the marrow is drawn into the syringe. Sometimes a small core of marrow is needed (a trephine biopsy) and this takes a few minutes longer.

This test can be done on the ward or in the out-patients department. When the local anaesthetic wears off you may feel an ache which can last for a few days.

Further tests

A chest x-ray is usually taken. Occasionally, if there is any doubt about the diagnosis, it may be necessary to remove an enlarged lymph gland to look at the cells under the microscope. This operation is called a lymph gland biopsy and may be done under a local or general anaesthetic.

What types of treatment are used?

Some people with chronic lymphocytic leukaemia never require any treatment at all if the illness is not causing any symptoms and is progressing only very slowly. Treatment is only started when the symptoms are becoming troublesome.

When treatment becomes necessary, you will be started on either tablets or intravenous chemotherapy.

If you have any questions, don't be afraid to ask your doctor or the nurse looking after you. It often helps to make a list of questions for your doctor and to take a friend or relative with you.

Some people find it reassuring to have another medical opinion to help them decide about their treatment. Most doctors will be pleased to refer you to another specialist for a second opinion if you feel this will be helpful.

Chemotherapy

Chemotherapy is the use of anti-cancer (cytotoxic) drugs which work by stopping the leukaemia cells from multiplying. The drugs circulate in the blood and can therefore reach leukaemia cells all over the body.

The drugs used to treat chronic lymphocytic leukaemia are usually given as tablets, and have few, if any, side effects. They may be given daily, over a period of time, or for a few days each month. The dose may be altered according to the results of your regular blood tests.

Treatment will be stopped if your blood count goes too low (i.e. if the white cell count or platelet count falls below a certain level) and then restarted.

Some people need stronger or different treatment, which is given intravenously, and steroids (Prednisone, Prednisolone) may sometimes be used, particularly if the level of haemoglobin in the blood falls very quickly. This is called 'haemolysis' and means that the red blood cells are being destroyed inappropriately by the spleen. This does not happen to everyone with CLL and usually only happens if you have an infection. If, at any point, you suddenly notice you are very tired or short of breath, contact the hospital immediately. The situation can be put right but don't delay getting in touch; it is much easier to deal with haemolysis early, rather than when you have become severely anaemic.

If at any time you notice anything else untoward happening, in particular, if you develop a temperature or any other signs of infection, again contact the hospital straight away. You may need to be admitted for intravenous antibiotics. Another infection which people with CLL can get is shingles. This is a virus infection which causes a painful red skin rash made up of little blisters. It often occurs round the chest but can involve any area of the body. If you think you may have shingles, contact your GP or the hospital immediately.

Side effects

The tablets used to treat chronic lymphocytic leukaemia do not usually have any side effects but may cause mild nausea, or, rarely, a rash.

Some of the intravenous drugs can cause other side effects such as nausea and vomiting, but you will be given anti-sickness drugs (anti-emetics) by the hospital doctor or your GP. Some of these chemotherapy drugs can make your mouth sore and cause small ulcers. Regular mouthwashes are important and the nurse will show you how to do these properly. If you don't feel like eating during treatment, you could try replacing some meals with nutritious drinks or a soft diet — BACUP's diet booklet *Diet and the Cancer Patient* has some useful tips on coping with eating problems.

Unfortunately, hair loss is another common side effect of the intravenous drugs. However, whether or not you lose your hair depends on the exact type of drugs you are receiving. It is best to ask your doctor what to expect.

People who do lose their hair often wear wigs, hats or scarves. Most in-patients are entitled to a free wig from the National Health Service and your doctor or the nurse looking after you will be able to arrange for a wig specialist to visit you. Although they may be hard to bear at the time, these side effects will disappear once your treatment is over, and if you do lose your hair it will grow back surprisingly quickly. BACUP has a booklet called *Coping With Hair Loss* which we would be happy to send you.

Chemotherapy affects people in different ways. Some people receiving the intravenous chemotherapy find they are able to lead a fairly normal life during their treatment, but many find they become very tired and have to take things much more slowly. Just do as much as you feel like and try not to overdo it.

Steroids

As mentioned above, steroids may be given as part of the treatment, usually only for a short period so that they have relatively few side effects but you may notice that you have a bigger appetite than usual, that you feel more energetic and have some difficulty in getting to sleep.

If you do need to take steroids for a longer period, you may have other temporary side effects which can include mild water retention, high blood pressure and a slightly greater risk of getting infections. You may also develop a high level of sugar in the blood; if this happens, your doctor will prescribe treatment which will need to be taken daily to bring the blood sugar level back to normal. You may need to do a simple test to check for sugar in your urine; the nurse will show you how to do this.

It is unusual for people with CLL to have to take steroids for a long time but if you do, you may also put on weight, especially around your face, waist and shoulders. It is important to remember that all these side effects are temporary and will gradually disappear as the steroid dose is reduced.

Effect on the blood count

Common to all of the cytotoxic drugs that are used for CLL is the fact that the drugs 'can't tell the difference' between a normal bone marrow cell that is dividing and a leukaemia cell. Chemotherapy can therefore, temporarily, reduce the number of normal cells in the blood. Whilst you are having treatment you will have regular blood tests to check that you have not become anaemic, but if this does happen, you will be given a blood transfusion. Sometimes the level of normal white cells can become very low, making you more susceptible to infection. As mentioned above, if you do get a temperature or any other sign of infection, you will need treatment with antibiotics and may need to be admitted to hospital. The drugs can also make the level of platelets low; if you notice bruising or any bleeding, contact the hospital immediately.

New treatment

A new drug, fludarabine, is currently being tested, with encouraging results, in people who are no longer responding to conventional treatment.

Follow up

CLL is an illness which you can have for a long time. It cannot be completely eradicated but treatment these days is effective and can keep the disease under control for years.

When your treatment has been completed, you will need to have regular check-ups and blood tests at the hospital. If you have any problems, or notice any new symptoms in between these times, let your doctor know as soon as possible.

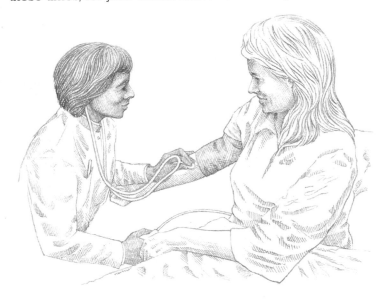

For more information about radiotherapy, chemotherapy, diet hints and hair loss, see our list of BACUP publications at the back of this booklet.

Research — clinical trials

Cancer doctors (oncologists) are continually looking for new treatments for CLL. If early work suggests that a new treatment might be more effective than the standard treatment, a clinical trial will be carried out to compare the new treatment with the currently available ones. Often several hospitals around the country take part in these trials.

So that the treatments may be accurately compared, a randomised study is usually done. This means that the treatment a patient receives is decided at random and not by the doctor treating the patient. This is because it has been shown that if a doctor (or patient) chooses the treatment, either may unintentionally bias the result of the trial.

In a randomised controlled clinical trial, half the patients will receive the best standard treatment and the other half will receive the new treatment. A treatment is deemed to be better either because it is more effective against the leukaemia or because it is equally effective and has the advantage of fewer unpleasant side effects.

Your doctor must have your informed consent before entering you into any clinical trial. This means that you know what the trial is about, you understand why it is being conducted and why you have been invited to take part, and the treatment has been discussed with you.

Even after agreeing to take part in a trial, you can still withdraw at any stage if you change your mind. Your decision will in no way affect your doctor's attitude towards you. If you choose not to take part or you withdraw from a trial, you will then receive the best standard treatment rather than the new one with which it is being compared.

If you do choose to take part in these trials, it is important to remember that whatever treatment you receive will have been carefully researched in preliminary studies, before it is fully tested in any randomised controlled clinical trial. By taking part in a trial you will also be helping to advance medical science and thus improve prospects for patients in the future.

Your feelings

Chronic lymphocytic leukaemia usually progresses very slowly and many people with the disease find that it does not affect their lives at all. However, for other people the mere mention of the word 'leukaemia' may cause great distress and they may feel completely overwhelmed by their emotions.

Some people never need any treatment for CLL and others may not need treatment for a long time. It can be very difficult to accept that you have a cancer and that nothing is beind done about it. Tell your doctor about your feelings so that he or she can explain to you why you don't actually need any treatment at that time.

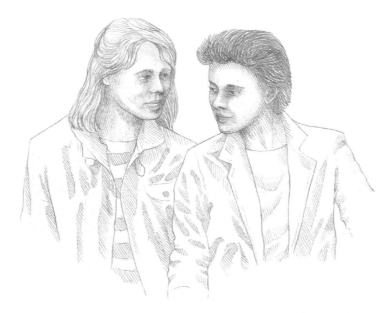

Many people experience a number of different emotions which can cause confusion and frequent changes of mood. You might not experience all the feelings discussed below or experience them in the same order. This does not mean, however, that you are not coping with your illness. Reactions differ from one person to another — there is no right or wrong way to feel. These emotions are part of the process that many people go through in trying to come to terms with their illness. Partners, family members and friends often experience similar feelings and frequently need as much support and guidance in coping with their feelings as you do.

Shock and disbelief

'I can't believe it' 'It can't be true'

This is often the immediate reaction when someone is told they have chronic lymphocytic leukaemia because of the frightening sound of the word 'leukaemia'. Even though your doctor tells you that this type of leukaemia is very mild, you may feel it hard to believe after all you may have read or heard about leukaemia in the past.

You may feel numb, unable to believe what is happening or to express any emotion. You may find that you can take in only a small amount of information and so you have to keep asking the same questions over and over again, or you need to be told the same bits of information repeatedly. This need for repetition is a common reaction to shock. Some people may find their feelings of disbelief make it difficult for them to talk about their illness with their family and friends, while others feel an overwhelming urge to discuss it with those around them; this may be a way of helping them to accept the news themselves.

Fear and uncertainty

'Am I going to die?' 'Will I be in pain?'

Leukaemia is a frightening word surrounded by fears and myths. One of the greatest fears expressed by almost all newly-diagnosed leukaemia patients is: 'Am I going to die?'

In fact, modern treatments mean that the disease can often be controlled for years and many patients can live an almost normal life.

'Will I be in pain?' and 'Will any pain be unbearable?' are other common fears. In fact, many leukaemia patients experience no pain at all. For those who do, there are many modern drugs which are very successful at relieving pain or keeping it under control.

Many people are anxious about their treatment; whether or not it will work and how to cope with possible side effects. It is best to discuss your individual treatment in detail with your doctor. Make a list of questions you may want to ask and don't be afraid to ask your doctor to repeat any answers or explanations you don't understand. You may like to take a close friend or relative to the appointment with you. If you are feeling upset, they may be able to remember details of the consultation which you might have forgotten or you may want them to ask some of the questions you yourself might be hesitant of putting to the doctor. Some people are afraid of the hospital itself. It can be a frightening place, especially if you have never been in one before, but talk about your fears to your doctor; he or she should be able to reassure you.

Often you will find that doctors may be unable to answer your questions fully, or that their answers may sound vague. It is often impossible to say for certain that the leukaemia has been totally eradicated. Doctors know from past experience approximately how many people will benefit from a certain treatment, but it is impossible to predict the future for individual people. Many people find this uncertainty hard to live with; not knowing whether or not you are cured can be disturbing.

Uncertainty about the future can cause a lot of tension, but fears and fantasies are often worse than the reality. Fear of the unknown can be terrifying, so acquiring some knowledge about your illness can be reassuring and discussing your findings with your family and friends can help to relieve tension caused by unnecessary worry.

Denial

'There's nothing really wrong with me' 'I haven't got cancer'

For many people, not wanting to know anything about their leukaemia, or wishing to talk as little as possible about it, is the best way of coping with the situation. If that's the way you feel, then just say quite firmly to the people around you that you would prefer not to talk about your illness, at least for the time being.

Sometimes, however, it is the other way round. You may find that it is your family and friends who are denying your illness. They appear to ignore the fact that you have leukaemia, perhaps by playing down your anxieties and symptoms or deliberately changing the subject. If this upsets or hurts you because you want them to support you by sharing what you feel, try telling them how you feel. Start perhaps by reassuring them that you do know what is happening and that it will help you if you can talk to them about your illness.

Anger

'Why me of all people?' 'And why right now?'

Anger can hide other feelings such as fear or sadness and you may vent your anger on those who are closest to you and on the doctors and nurses who are caring for you. If you hold religious beliefs you may feel angry with your God.

It is understandable that you may be deeply upset by many aspects of your illness and you should not feel guilty about your angry thoughts or irritable moods. However, relatives and friends may not always realise that your anger is really directed at your illness and not against them. If you can, it may be helpful to tell them this at a time when you are not feeling quite so angry, or if you would find that difficult, perhaps you could show them this section of the booklet. If you are finding it difficult to talk to your family it may help to discuss the situation with a trained counsellor or psychologist. BACUP can give you details of how to get this sort of help in your area (see page 24).

Blame and guilt

'If I hadn't...this would never have happened'

Sometimes people blame themselves or other people for their illness, trying to find reasons why it should have happened to them. This may be because we often feel better if we know why something has happened, but since doctors rarely know exactly what has caused an individual's cancer, there's no reason for you to blame yourself.

Resentment

'It's all right for you, you haven't got to put up with this'

Understandably, you may be feeling resentful and miserable because you have cancer while other people are well. Similar feelings of resentment may crop up from time to time during the course of your illness and treatment for a variety of reasons. Relatives too can sometimes resent the changes that the patient's illness makes to their lives.

It is usually helpful to bring these feelings out into the open so that they can be aired and discussed. Bottling up resentment can make everyone feel angry and guilty.

Withdrawal and isolation

'Please leave me alone'

There may be times during your illness when you want to be left alone to sort out your thoughts and emotions. This can be hard for your family and friends who want to share this difficult time with you. It will make it easier for them to cope however, if you reassure them that although you may not feel like discussing your illness at the moment, you will talk to them about it when you are ready.

Sometimes an unwillingness to talk can be caused by depression. It may be an idea to discuss this with your GP who can prescribe a course of antidepressant drugs or refer you to a doctor who specialises in the emotional problems of cancer patients.

Learning to cope

After any treatment for cancer it can take a long time to come to terms with your emotions. Not only do you have to cope with the knowledge that you have cancer but also the physical effects of the treatment.

The treatment for leukaemia can cause unpleasant side effects but some people do manage to lead an almost normal life during their treatment. Obviously you will need to take time off for your actual treatment and some time afterwards to recover. Just do as much as you feel like and try to get plenty of rest.

Don't see it as a sign of failure if you have not been able to cope on your own. Once other people understand how you are feeling they can be more supportive.

Who and what to tell

Some families find it difficult to talk about leukaemia or share their feelings. The first reaction of many relatives is that the patient should not be told he or she has leukaemia. They may be afraid that the patient will be unable to cope with the news. If a decision is made not to tell, the family then has to cover up and hide information. These secrets within a family can be very difficult to keep and they can isolate the patient. They make him or her more frightened and can cause tension between family members. In any case, many people suspect their diagnosis, even if they are not actually told.

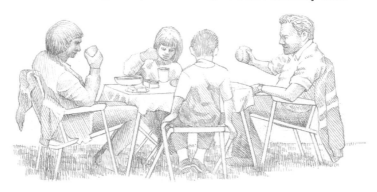

Whether you are the patient or a close relative, look out for friends and relatives with a positive attitude as they are always more helpful than gloomy, pessimistic ones.

Relatives and friends can help by listening carefully to what, and how much, the patient wants to say. Don't rush into talking about the illness. Often it is enough just to listen and let the patient talk when he or she is ready.

Talking to children

Deciding what to tell your children about your leukaemia is difficult. How much you tell them will depend upon their age and how grown up they are. Very young children are concerned with immediate events. They don't understand illness and need only simple explanations of why their relative or friend has had to go into hospital or isn't his or her normal self. Slightly older children may understand a story explanation in terms of good cells and bad cells but all children need to be repeatedly reassured that your illness is not their fault because, whether they show it or not, children often feel they may somehow be to blame and may feel guilty for a long time. Most children of about 10 years old and over can grasp fairly complicated explanations.

Adolescents may find it particularly difficult to cope with the situation because they feel they are being forced back into the family just as they were beginning to break free and gain their independence.

An open, honest approach is usually the best way for all children. Listen to their fears and be aware of any changes in their behaviour. This may be their way of expressing their feelings. It may be better to start by giving only small amounts of information and gradually building up a picture of your illness. Even very young children can sense when something is wrong, so don't keep them in the dark about what is going on. Their fears of what it might be are likely to be far worse than the reality.

What you can do

A lot of people feel helpless when they are first told they have cancer and think there is nothing they can do, other than hand themselves over to doctors and hospitals. This is not so. There are many things you, and your family, can do at this time.

Understanding your illness

If you and your family understand your illness and its treatment you will be better prepared to cope with the situation. In this way you at least have some idea of what you are facing.

However, for information to be of value it must come from a reliable source to prevent it causing unnecessary fears. Personal medical information should come from your own doctor who is familiar with your medical background. As mentioned earlier, it can be useful to make a list of questions before your visit or take a friend or relative with you to remind you of things you want to know but can forget so easily. Other sources of information are given at the end of this booklet.

Practical and positive tasks

At times you may not be able to do things you used to take for granted. But as you begin to feel better you can set yourself some simple goals and gradually build up your confidence. Take things slowly and one step at a time.

Many people talk about 'fighting their illness'. This is a healthy response and you can do it by becoming involved in your illness. One easy way of doing this is by planning a healthy, well-balanced diet. Another way is to learn relaxation techniques which you can practise at home with tapes. Contact BACUP for more information.

Many people find it helpful to take some regular exercise. The type of exercise you take, and how strenuous, depends on what you are used to and how well you feel. Set yourself realistic aims and build up slowly.

Who can help?

The most important thing to remember is that there are people available to help you and your family. Often it is easier to talk to someone who is not directly involved with your illness. You may find it helpful to go to a counsellor, who is specially trained to listen and who will help you to talk about the things you are finding difficult to cope with or are causing you problems. BACUP runs a one-to-one counselling service in London, or can put you in touch with a counsellor in your area, see page 24 for more details.

Some people find great comfort in religion at this time and it may help for them to talk to a local minister, hospital chaplain or other religious leader. The nurses at BACUP are also happy to discuss any problems and they can put you in touch with a counsellor who lives near you or a local leukaemia support group.

There are several other people who can offer support in the community. District nurses work closely with GPs and make regular visits to some patients and their families at home. In many areas of the country there are also Macmillan and Marie Curie nurses, who are specially trained to look after people with leukaemia in their own homes. Let your GP know if you are having any problems so that proper home care can be arranged.

Some hospitals have their own emotional support services with specially trained staff and many of the nurses on the ward will have been given training in counselling as well as being able to give advice about practical problems. The hospital social worker is also often able to help in many ways including counselling and giving information about social services and other benefits you may be able to claim while you are ill. For example, you may be entitled to meals on wheels, a home help or hospital fares. The social worker may also be able to help arrange childcare during and after treatment and, if necessary, help with the cost of childminders.

But there are people who require more than advice and support. They may find that, despite their best efforts, the impact of leukaemia leads to depression, feelings of helplessness and anxiety. Specialist help in coping with these emotions is available in some hospitals. Ask your hospital consultant or GP to refer you to a doctor who is an expert in the special emotional problems of leukaemia patients and their relatives.

Sick pay and benefits

If you are employed, and unable to work, your employer will pay your first twenty-eight weeks' sick pay. If, after this period, you are still unable to work you can claim Invalidity Benefit from the Benefits Agency.

If you are unemployed and not fit to work you will need to switch from Unemployment Benefit to Sickness Benefit. To do this you should contact your local Benefits Agency office and arrange to send them regular sickness certificates from your doctor. If you are ill and not at work, do remember to ask your family doctor for a medical certificate to cover the period of your illness. If you are in hospital, ask the doctor or nurse for a certificate, which you will need to claim benefit.

If, because of your illness, you are finding it difficult to manage on your income, you may be entitled to Income Support (previously called Supplementary Benefit) and in some circumstances, you may be able to claim additional benefits.

For full advice on all the benefits available to you, contact your local Benefits Agency office, Citizens' Advice Bureau or Social Services office. Their addresses and telephone numbers are in the 'phone book.

BACUP's services

Cancer Information Service

This service is staffed by specially trained cancer nurses. If you ring or write to us, your phone call or letter will always be answered by a nurse who can give you information on all aspects of cancer and its treatment and who will offer practical and emotional support, whether you have cancer yourself, or are the friend or relative of someone with cancer. A computerised directory and a library of resources are used by the nurses to provide information to anyone who enquires about treatment, research, support groups, therapists, counsellors, financial assistance, insurance, home nursing services, and much more. The nurse can also send you any of our other booklets which might be helpful.

The Cancer Information Service is open to telephone enquiries from 10 am to 7 pm, Monday to Thursday, and until 5.30 pm on Friday. The number is 071 613 2121 if you are ringing from London. You can call the service free of charge from outside the 071 and 081 telephone districts on 0800 18 11 99.

Cancer Counselling Service

Emotional difficulties linked to cancer are not always easy to talk about and are often hardest to share with those to whom you are closest. Trained counsellors use their skills to help people talk about their thoughts, feelings and ideas and perhaps untangle some of the difficulties and confusion that living with cancer brings.

BACUP runs a one-to-one counselling service based at its London offices which it is intended to develop nationwide. The Counselling Service can also give you information about counselling services in your area, and discuss with you whether counselling would be appropriate and helpful. For more information about counselling, or to make an appointment with BACUP's Cancer Counselling Service, please ring 071 696 9000 between 10 am and 5 pm, Monday to Friday.

Other useful organisations

Leukaemia Research Fund
43 Great Ormond Street
London
WC1N 3JJ
Tel: 071 405 0101

Leukaemia Research Fund
  in Scotland
37 Whittinghame Drive
Glasgow G12 0YH
Tel: 041 339 1101

Devotes all its resources to research into the causes, treatment and cure of leukaemia, the lymphomas and myeloma. Provides a patient information service and booklets on the diseases and their treatment.

Leukaemia Care Society
14 Kingfisher Court
Venny Bridge
Pinhoe
Exeter
Devon EX4 8JN
Tel: 0392 464848

Groups throughout the United Kingdom. Offers support, befriending and companionship to patients and their families. Limited financial assistance is available and a small number of holiday caravans.

CancerLink
17 Britannia Street
London
WC1X 9JN
Tel: 071 833 2451

9 Castle Terrace
Edinburgh
EH1 2DP
Tel: 031 228 5557

Offers support and information on all aspects of cancer in response to telephone and letter enquiries. Acts as a resource to over 370 cancer support and self-help groups throughout the UK, and publishes a range of publications on issues about cancer.

Cancer Care Society
21 Zetland Road
Redland
Bristol
BS6 7AH
Tel: 0272 427419 or 0272 232302

Offers emotional support and practical help where possible through support groups around the country. Telephone and one-to-one counselling, telephone link service, holiday accommodation and information on other charities and cancer-related organisations.

Cancer Relief Macmillan Fund
15-19 Britten Street
London
SW3 3TZ
Tel: 071 351 7811

Provides home care nurses through the Macmillan Service and financial grants for people with cancer and their families.

Marie Curie Cancer Care
28 Belgrave Square
London
SW1X 8QG
Tel: 071 235 3325

Runs eleven centres (hospices) throughout the UK and a community nursing service which works with the district nursing service and supports cancer patients and their carers in their homes.

Tak Tent Cancer Support — Scotland
G Block
Western Infirmary
Glasgow
G11 6NT
Tel: 041 334 6699/041 357 4519

Offers emotional support and information to cancer patients, their relatives and friends and professional staff involved in their care. Network of support groups throughout Scotland.

Tenovus Cancer Information Centre
142 Whitchurch Road
Cardiff
CF4 3NA
Tel: 0222 691846 (Admin)
    0800 526527 (Freephone)

Provides an information service on all aspects of cancer. Operates a drop-in centre, helpline, and support groups.

The Ulster Cancer Foundation
40-42 Eglantine Avenue
Belfast
BT9 6DX
Tel: 0232 663439

Provides a cancer information helpline, resource centre and support groups for patients and relatives.

Recommended reading list

*Clyne Rachel
Cancer: Your Life, Your Choice
Wellingborough, Thorsons Publishing Group, 1989
(ISBN 0-7225-21-030)

Bryan, Jenny, Lyall, Joanna
Living with Cancer
Penguin 1987
(ISBN 0-14-009409-1)

Lynn, Joan
Cancer Treatment and Care: a guide for patients, families and carers
Northcote House, 1992
(ISBN 0-7463-0581-8)

Faulder, Carolyn
A Special Gift: The Story of Dr Vicky Clement-Jones and the Foundation of BACUP
London, Michael Joseph
(ISBN 0-7181-3442-7)

Kfir, Nira and Slevin, Maurice
Challenging Cancer: From Chaos to Control
London, Tavistock/Routledge
(ISBN 0-415-06344-2)

* Williams, Chris and Sue
Cancer: A guide for patients and their families
Chichester, Wiley, 1986
(ISBN 0-471-91017-1)

* These books are now out of print but may be available from libraries.